JOURNEY INTO TIMELESSNESS

Sylvia Talkington

Published by Simple Naturalist Books

Publishing assistance by BookCrafters, Parker, Colorado.
www.bookcrafters.net

Dedication

For my mother who was a writer and poet.
For my father who was a forest lover.

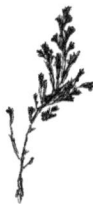

Introduction

IN AUTUMN 1981 I was desperate for time away from the normal craziness of a family and working full time in a hospital critical care unit. Growing up an only child I had no idea what to do with a three, four, five, and nine year old. They delighted me and exhausted me. During that year I'd also written the first *pocket guide* ever published.

George Lucas introduced us to Star Wars in 1977, taking us to a universe far, far away. *ECG-A Pocket Guide* was crafted from notes on paper scraps using a Selectric typewriter that sat on a vintage editor's desk. The desk also served as a rebel base for my very own Luke Skywalker, Leah Organa, and Han Solo. While they plotted overthrow of the evil Empire, I was plotting escape.

In May I'd ventured into the foreign universe of New York City at the request of a small publisher. Who knows, maybe it was the Force that kept me going at warp speed for months to achieve a dream. By October I was longing for sanctuary at a hidden outpost.

One Friday I left the Jedi in the care of a babysitter, whom they immediately declared Darth Vader. I had no idea where Taos, New Mexico was. I used the grocery money to buy a bus ticket thinking surely Taos must have a Holiday Inn. I knew it was in the mountains. Surely a stream or forest nearby where I could journal and paint. Peace and Quiet! A hungry rebel force greeted my husband who would be blind-sided by my defection. I posted a list of pre-made meals and snacks and left a note: *Be home Sunday night.*

Since that initial adventure I've returned thirty of thirty-six years; not to Taos, but a nearby place; Posi-Ouinge at Ojo Caliente NM. There, prehistoric peoples built ancient dwellings *above the place of the green bubbling springs*. Here, origin stories cross boundaries between then and now creating a place of mystical timelessness. On an open mesa overlooking a branch of the Rio Ojo, pottery shards are strewn on a clay landscape hidden by piñon and chamisa and scampered upon by striped lizards. Below the mesa, hot mineral waters refresh the soul as much as the body. Posi is suspended in seasons, below constellations and meteor showers in an inky black sky evoking a *galaxy far far away*.

S. T.
February 3, 2021

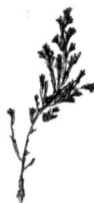

Preface

A JOURNEY IS AN UNEXPLAINABLE yearning to find, to discover, to know, to understand something. That *something* may be discovered in a physical or spiritual place; most often it's both. With each return to such a place a deeper and deeper communion satisfies with new discoveries. Along the way, memories and visions of that oneness embed themselves in our minds.

Posi-Ouinge is made of myth and legend. Its origin story is, like all oral and written history, a ballad of longing. A journey of searching for a home. In the mists of time unknown, prehistoric inhabitants emerged from a watery birthplace to travel from north to south as two separate groups. Both followed the source of life along waterways, then unnamed. One group went south along the Rio Chama; the other went south along the Rio Grande. These groups reunited at Posi-Ouinge in the Ojo Caliente drainage area. It has been a gathering place and source of healing for thousands of years. Posi was the largest of four villages in the area surrounding natural hot springs. In the 1880s, Archeologists Adolph Bandelier and Edgar Hewitt described the pueblo's layout as a structure with possibly a thousand ground floor rooms topped by second and third levels. These prehistoric peoples are ancestors of today's Native American Rio Grande and Tewa tribes. The poems that follow have been selected from writings representing thirty of thirty-six years of pilgrimage to Posi. For insight into the poems see End Notes.

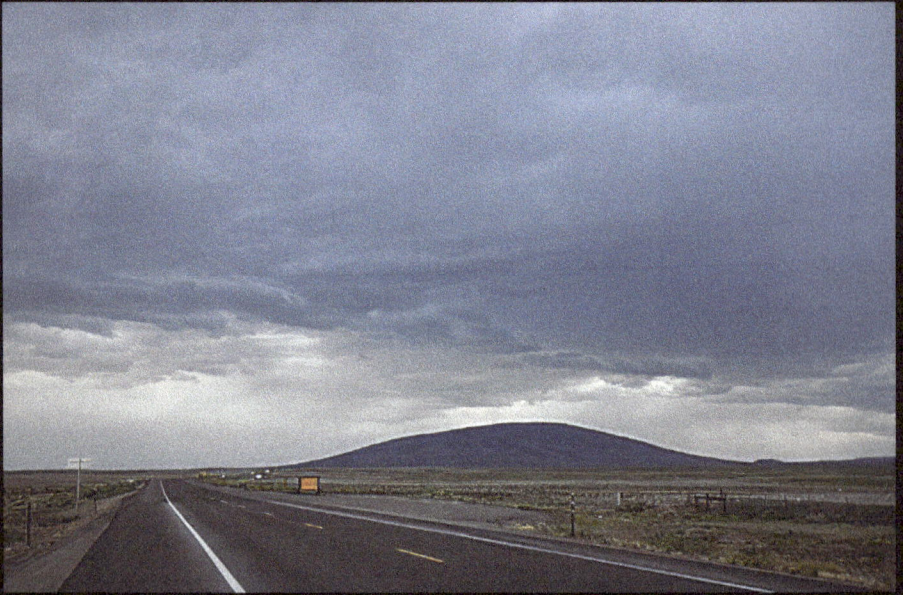

RETURN

By GPS reckoning Ojo Caliente is 317.9 miles south of my home. When I turn south at Antonito (mile 258.) San Antonio Mountain, a 10,908 ft monolithic mound dominates the Taos Plateau volcanic field. From that location it guards the entrance to sacred ground. San Antonio Mountain is woven into the cosmology and mythology of the Tewa-speaking peoples of the Rio Grande Valley. As I continue to drive south on a moonscape of volcanic detritus it becomes a land of mirages. Were the first people comforted by optical illusions of water ahead?

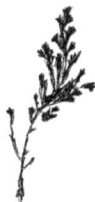

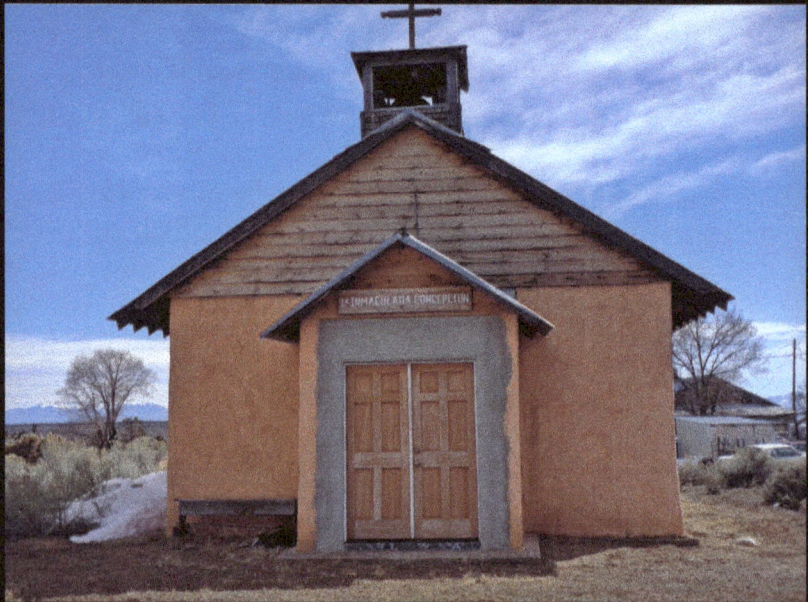

At Tres Piedras I pull off beside a silent and shuttered adobe church where yucca entice moths and blooming cacti lure shutterbugs. It has become a ritual to pray here. Did the prehistoric peoples pray here for direction and reassurance as I do? I persevere on as they did.

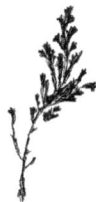

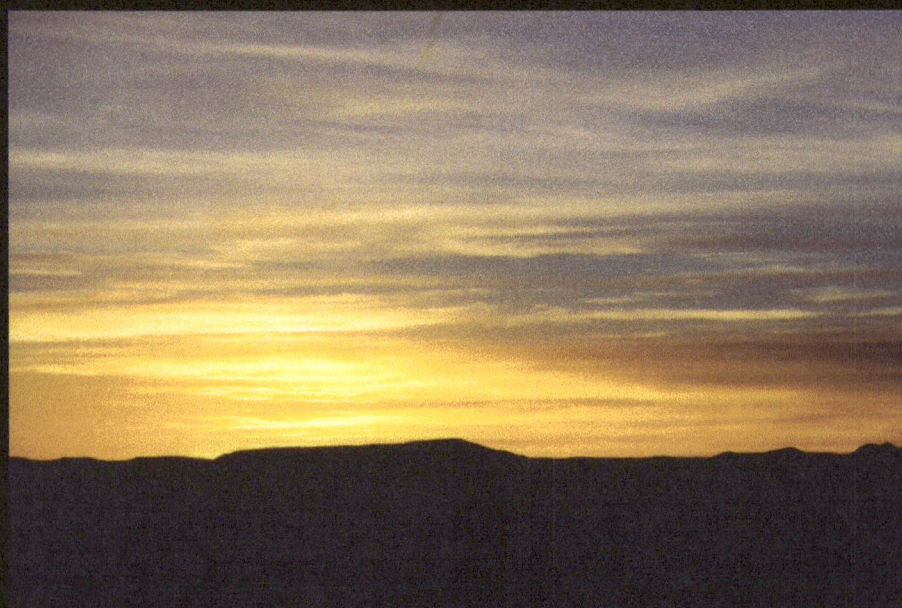

ARRIVAL AT A DESTINATION

Always a long-anticipated reunion.
Soaked in memories,
Wrapped in herbal promises,
Floating on waters of iron, lithium, arsenic, soda.
Gentle reminders of emergences past, present and to come.

I have always been of
Vast distances of sky and land,
Mountain silhouettes,
Cottonwood trees on coursing water,
White dirt and red mud,
Fields of blue corn,
I am Summer People and I am Home.

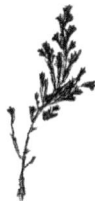

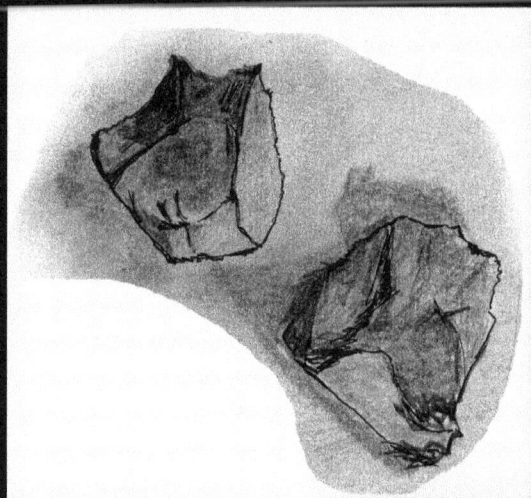
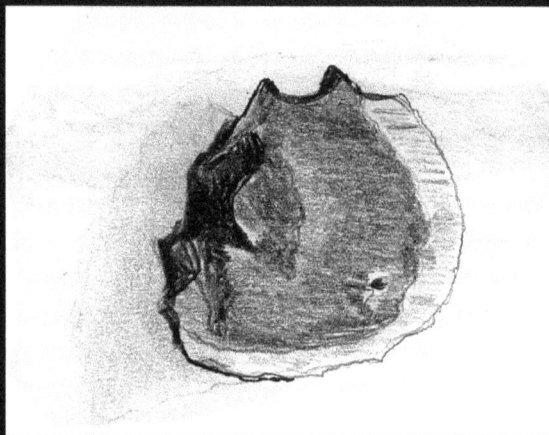
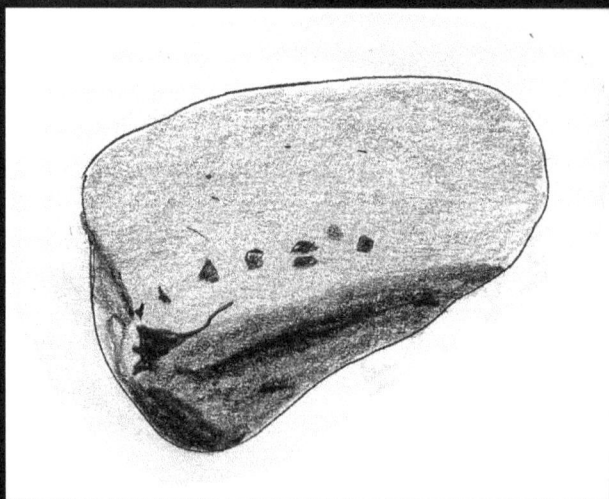

A SACRED PLACE

Today I welcomed the sun and was filled with gratitude. For being alive in a holy place where relics enshrine Tewa origins and southward migrations. This place marking a reunion of Summer and Winter People.

Black on white pottery fragments hide below piñons in white and red mesa dust.

A lone flint scraper reveals a perfectly notched thumbprint. Obsidian chips echo a mountain birth.

Among the relics I am humbled.

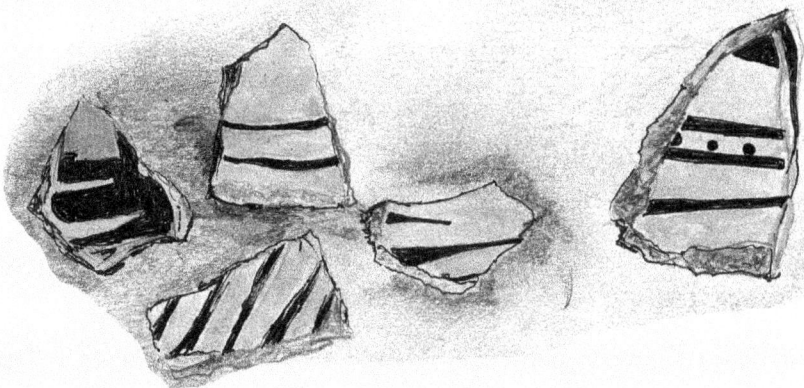

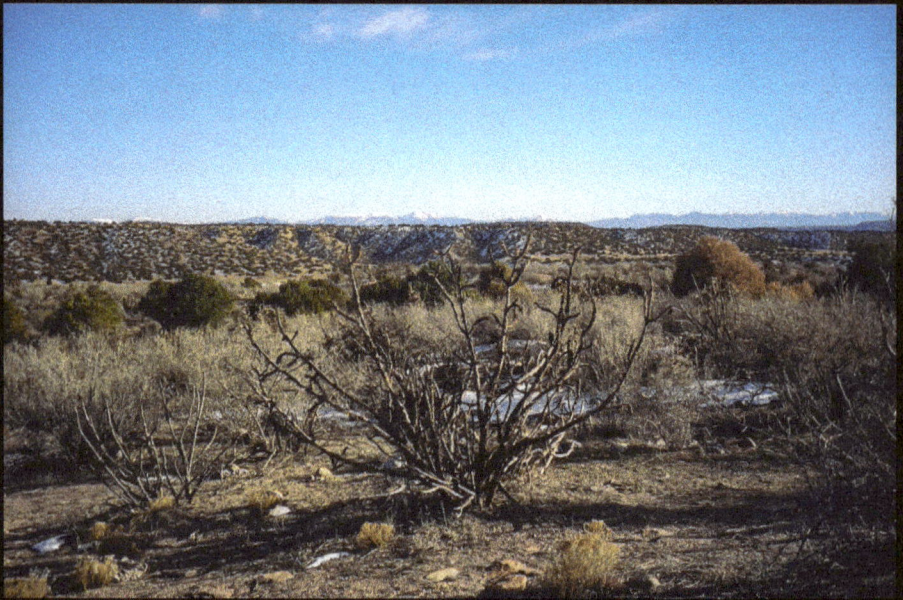

MESSAGES

What messages are scattered here where I am roaming?
What stories are told?
Posi residents.
Summer and Winter people together.
Sitting in warm sun.
Creating earthen pots.
Vessels for storing and cooking.
Black lines on white clay.
Clues of a distant past.

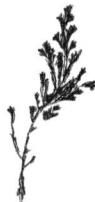

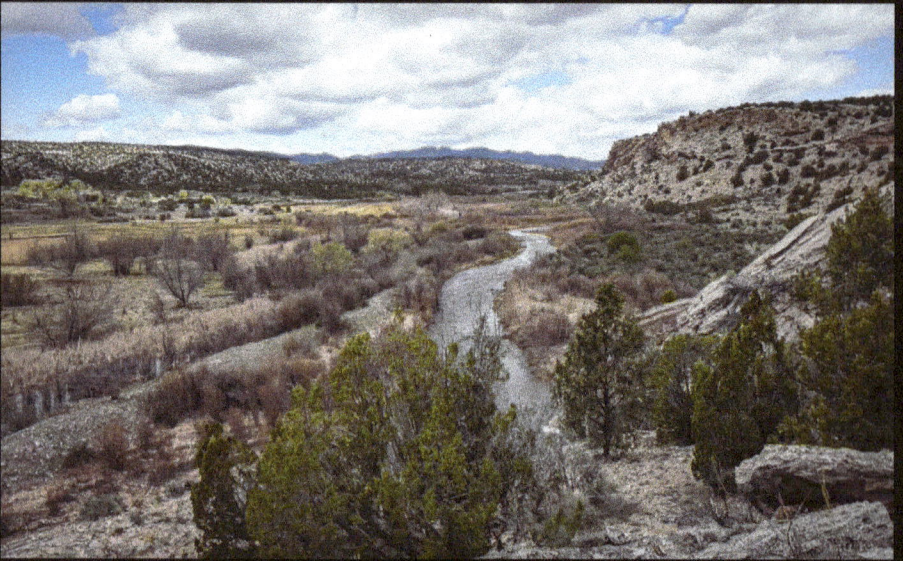

A LANDSCAPE OF SEASONS

Four seasons create a timeless landscape of a place and a people defined by water and earth.

WATER

Winter
Rio Ojo flows lazily and gently,
pushed along by seeping hot mineral water.
Mini icebergs wander
Downstream.

Spring
Rio Ojo flows hastily and urgently,
forced along to hungry apple green fields.
Fast currents rush nourishment
Downstream.

Summer
Rio Ojo flows seriously and secretively,
compelled by heat that sizzles the brain.
Hidden eddies send welcome relief
Downstream.

Autumn
Rio Ojo flows benevolently and gracefully,
motivated by a sense of fullness.
Auburn leaves pirouette, without hurry, to die
Downstream.

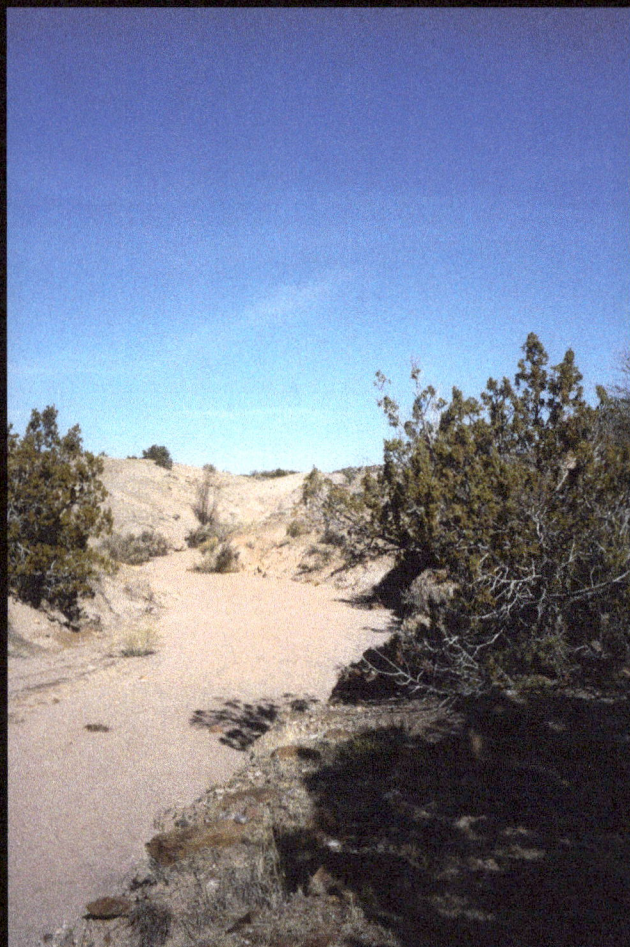

EARTH

Winter
Quiet time descends upon the landscape.
Go silently say Spirits.
Along snow covered paths
Onto sacred ground.

Spring
Celebration blooms upon the landscape.
Go expectantly say Spirits.
Through yellow, red, orange cacti
Onto sacred ground.

Summer
Midday sun preys upon the landscape.
Go carefully say Spirits.
Over baked arroyos where whiptails play
Onto sacred ground.

Autumn
Amber glow hazes upon the landscape.
Go with thanksgiving say Spirits.
To waiting mineral pools below red clay turrets
Into sacred waters.

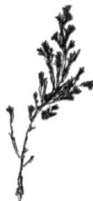

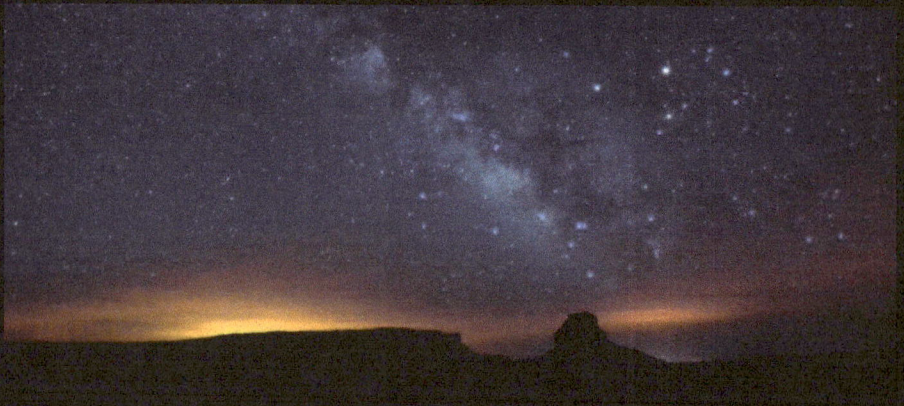

A LANDSCAPE OF SKY

Days and nights create a timeless skyscape defined by sun and moon, planets, and constellations.

Sunrise

Does not creep up on earth in dullness here.
It makes a flaming crimson appearance on the eastern horizon.

Declaring the certainty of another day.

Day

From sacred mountain to sacred mountain a day unfolds with grandeur from chill morning to cool evening in this land of many moods.

Sunset

It is impossible to go indoors. I am watching for sunset.

Transformed into a stone in a circle of rocks,
I sit wrapped in a warm herbal blanket.
Scent of piñon and sage wafts from the firepit.
Opalescent pinks will soon color a winter sky.
I find a patience, normally unknown and rarely practiced.
A tranquility that eases day into night.

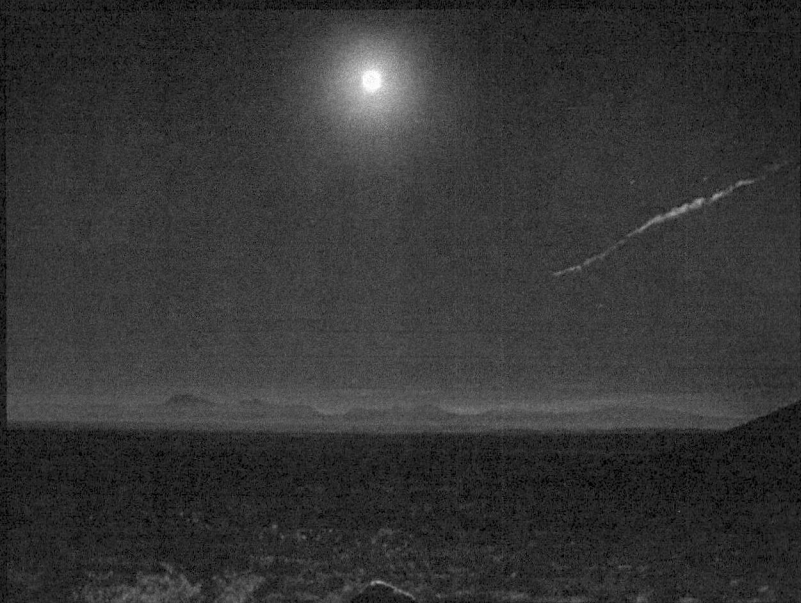

Night

Planets rise and set above ghostly ruins.
Meteor showers chase among constellations.
Quadrantids in Winter.
Perseids in Summer.
On a high mesa I lay on my back.
Arms under my head.
Zooming Perseids
Shoot star stuff into the black above me.

Moon

I have never been alone here at Ojo.
Spirits travel with me to this place.
I climb a rocky trail in ambient light.
Rocks twinkle under-foot.
Mimicking the Milky Way.
My footsteps sure and true
in half moon's glow.

Phases of the moon influence my days as if I were a tide.
On these recurring journeys to this magical place
I become nocturnal.
A bat soaring in and out of an ancient pueblo.

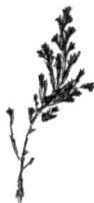

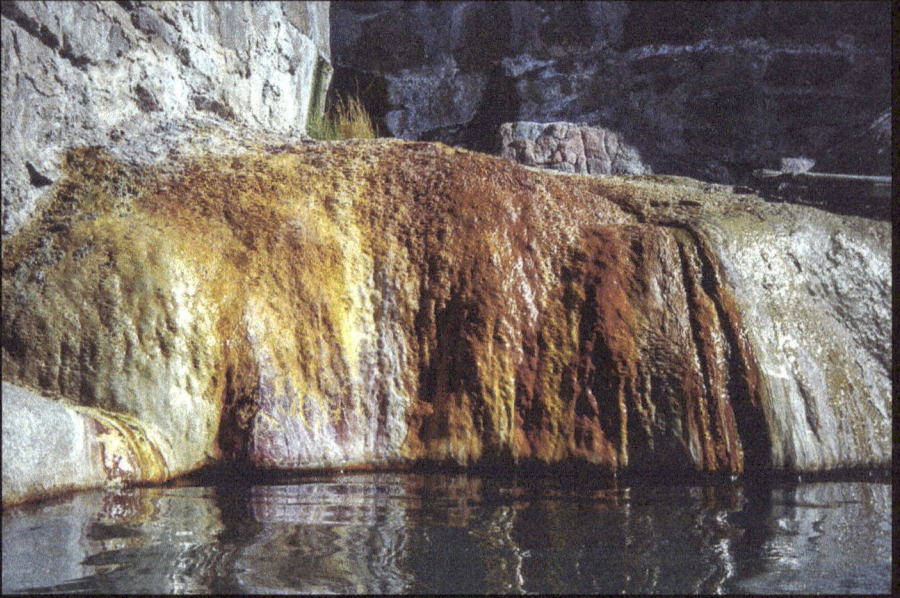

A LANDSCAPE OF TIME

Time stops and retraces itself here

Today moves along a path of antiquities
born of yesterdays.

Tomorrow forms from ancient waters bathing clay.
Mud of rocks undoing.
Forming murky pools.
Fulfilling the destiny of millennia.

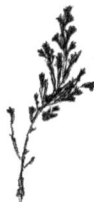

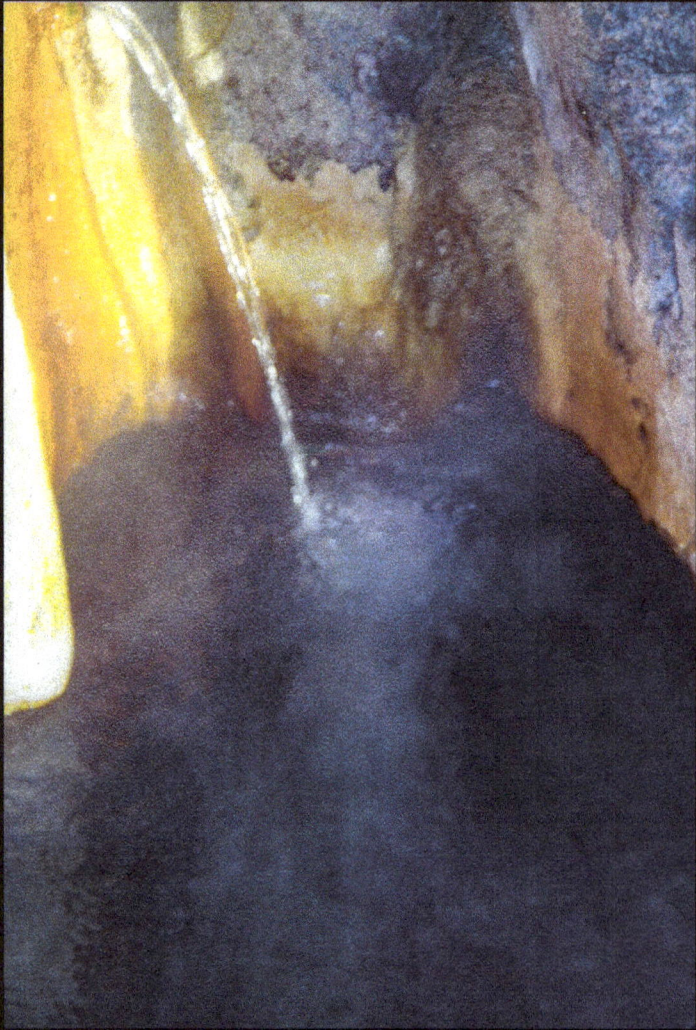

EMERGENCE

Ancient rocks and mud chant around me.
"Come into the world of your beginning."

I submit and submerge below the surface of the pool.
Amphibious skin and primordial gills
seem to mysteriously reappear.

Effervescent blurbles emerge from the depths
Forming concentric circles across the surface.
Emitting fragrances of iron, soda, lithium, and arsenic.

I enclose myself in a hidden red rock cleft.
Perpetually flowing iron water pours over the top of my head
Coursing down over my shoulders and between my breasts.

I stretch my legs.
Thankful for these pilgrimages
Where I discover a renewed strength for walking.

My body simmers in a geothermal broth.
Aches stew into mineral relief.
Aging muscles soak to rejuvenation.

My psyche spirals up in a dwarf tornado of mist.
Anxieties vaporize into sulfurous retreat.
Youthful affirmations soak my mind to restoration.

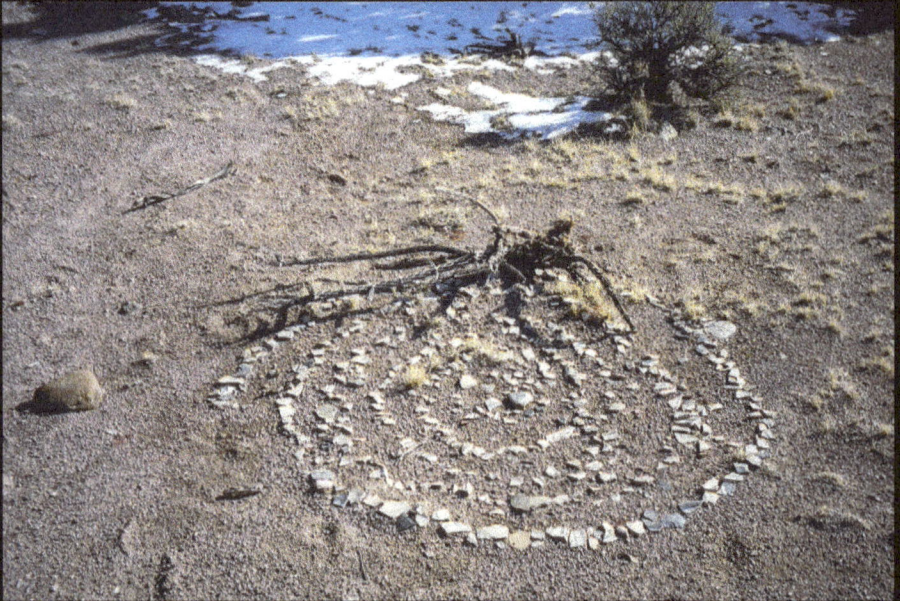

SPIRAL OF LIFE

A stone spiral on the plateau is replicated in a broom swept
courtyard. At dawn and moonrise I walk the spiral as a ritual of
reunion and re-emergence.

Walking the spiral path slowly in silence.
I am alone with my thoughts.

At the Center, I re-collect who I am.
My origins.

I recall what gives me strength when the outer world challenges
and wears.

That is why I come to Ojo, to Posi.
They bring me close to my beginnings.

My challenge is to face reality in the temporal world.
Without forgetting.
I am creature of primordial beginnings.
Water, Earth, and Sky.
Rock Collector, Forest Lover, Desert Wanderer.
Sun Chaser, Moon Writer, Star Watcher.
Bound eternally to Nature.
The life spiral reminds me that every new adventure begins from
a previous journey.

We must begin at the end of that journey to discover a new
beginning.

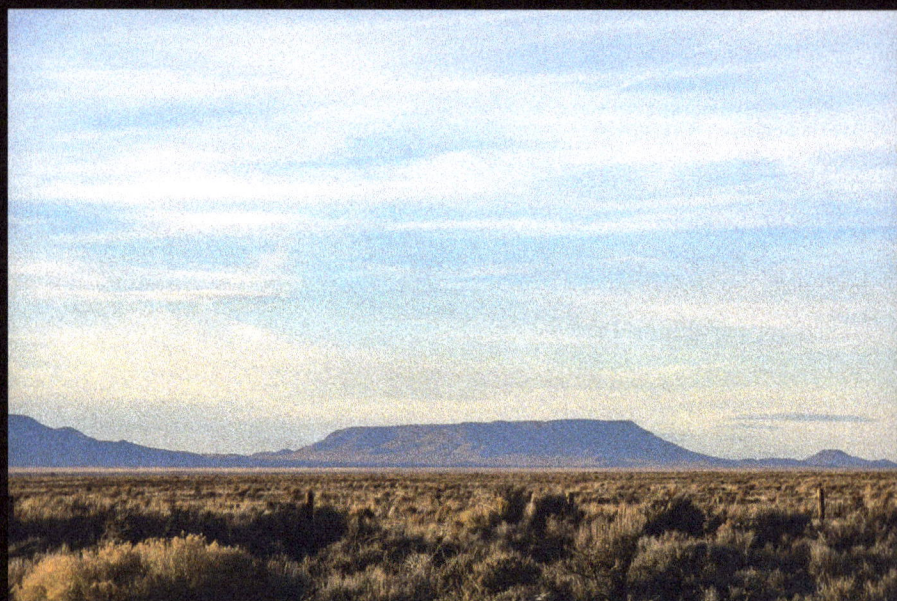

RETURN TO THE WORLD

Here, I am a child of the Earth.
Here, I am far from the World.
Here, I find strength and peace to return to the world.
To follow Life's Spiral.

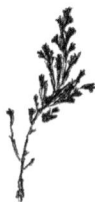

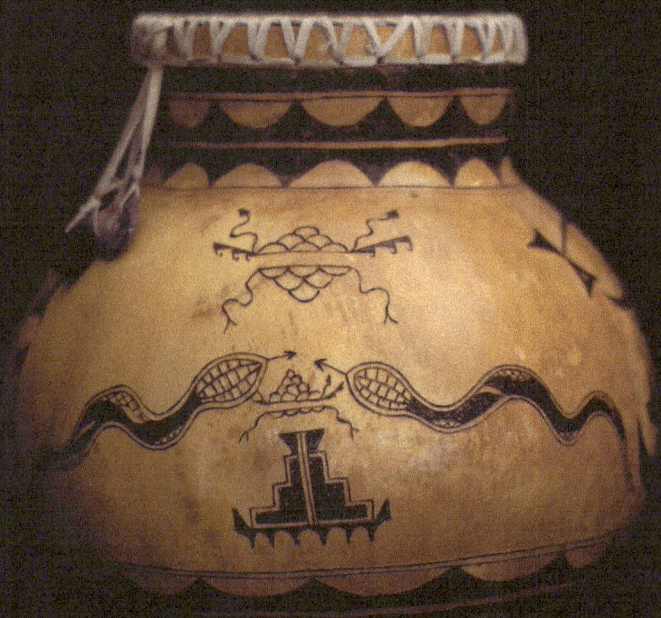

End notes:

Tewa Origin and Migration myths

The Tewa were living in a world under a sandy lake far to the north. It was a dark world of supernaturals, men, and animals. Among the supernaturals were two mothers for all the Tewa; Blue Corn Woman – or Summer Mother and White Corn Maiden or Winter Mother. They asked one of the men to explore a way for the people to leave the lake. His first attempt was to the north. He saw only mist and haze. The next three attempts were to the west, south, and east. He found only mist and haze. He reported he had seen nothing; the world was "ochu"- green or unripe. Next, he was asked to go to the above where he came upon an open space. All the predatory animals were gathered. They gave him a bow, arrows, and quiver and dressed him in buckskin. When he returned, the waiting people knew they'd been accepted by the animals into the open space above. Thus, the migration out of the lake began. Summer People followed one route. Winter People followed another. On their way they made twelve stops. At the twelfth stop the two groups reunited and founded a village called Posi,-Ouinge near present day Ojo Caliente. Summer and Winter people remained together.

For more information see the acclaimed work by social anthropologist Alphonso Ortiz; The Tewa World – Space, Time, Being & Becoming in a Pueblo Society. 1969.

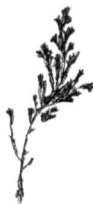

ACKNOWLEDGEMENTS

Special thank you to William Knoll, photographer, who gifted me with his time by scanning my original photographs and illustrations; photographing San Ildefonso red clay pottery with serpent design. And, Tim Kathka, photographer, who provided resizing of several additional photographs.

All photos were taken at the time of a return to Ojo Caliente with the exception of the following:

San Antonio Mountain - Page 5 - NM Bureau of Tourism.

Rio Ojo – Page 14 – Open source, stock photo without credit.

Night Sky – Page 18 – Corrie Photography 2014.

NM True Dark Skies Trail - Page 20 - NM Tourism Department.

Gourd with etched Tewa symbols - page 30 Bill Beekkman - Artisan and Flintknapper.

Avanyou – Tewa Water Spirit - red clay pot.
Potter – Geraldine Gutierrez, San Ildefonso Pueblo, NM
Purchase date unknown. 1980s

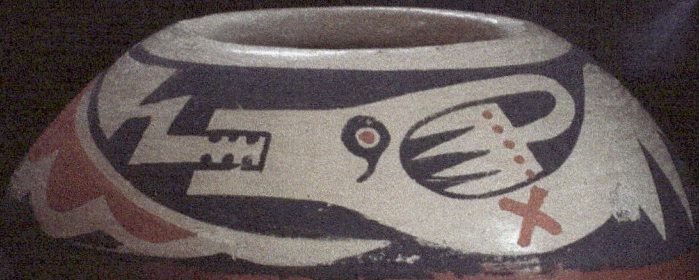

www.ingramcontent.com/pod-product-compliance
Lightning Source LLC
Chambersburg PA
CBHW052125030426

42335CB00025B/3113